Rhinitis

Management Guidelines

THIRD EDITION

BRITISH SOCIETY FOR ALLERGY
AND CLINICAL IMMUNOLOGY
ENT Sub-Committee

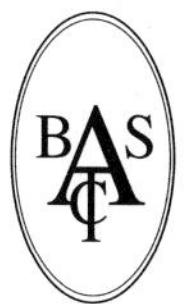

MARTIN DUNITZ

- *Skin prick testing is safe, inexpensive and helps the clinician to make a diagnosis as well as graphically demonstrating the problem to the patient.*

- *Allergen avoidance, in particular of house dust mite when this is responsible in perennial rhinitis, may be helpful.*

- *Antihistamines often help the symptoms of sneezing and itchy eyes.*

- *Topical nasal steroids work well for all symptoms including blockage in persistent allergic rhinitis.*

- *Compliance and the continued use of topical nasal steroids are crucial to maintain symptomatic control in persistent allergic rhinitis.*

- *Unilateral nasal polyps or mucopurulent discharge are symptoms which are a cause for concern and warrant referral.*

Foreword

Rhinitis is an under-appreciated cause of morbidity which imposes heavy costs on sufferers. Symptoms resemble those of a severe cold and are often permanent. The condition causes misery and underperformance which can, in some circumstances, cause sufferers to lose their jobs.

In addition, it is not always appreciated that rhinitis can have serious secondary effects, including sinusitis, and its contribution to the deterioration of lower airways function in asthma is only now beginning to be understood.

Fortunately the nose is simple to examine and allergic rhinitis is relatively easy to diagnose at primary care level. This is done by taking a careful history and performing simple skin prick tests.

Treatment measures are continually improving; recent additions to the range of topical corticosteroids have minimal potential for systemic effects, which make them useful in the treatment of children and asthmatics, in whom steroid overload may be a concern. Intranasal antihistamines have been introduced and better allergen avoidance measures developed, for example protective mattress covers.

This handbook has therefore been produced to help GPs identify and treat a debilitating and potentially serious disease.

Dr Glenis K. Scadding MA, MD, FRCP
Consultant Rhinologist

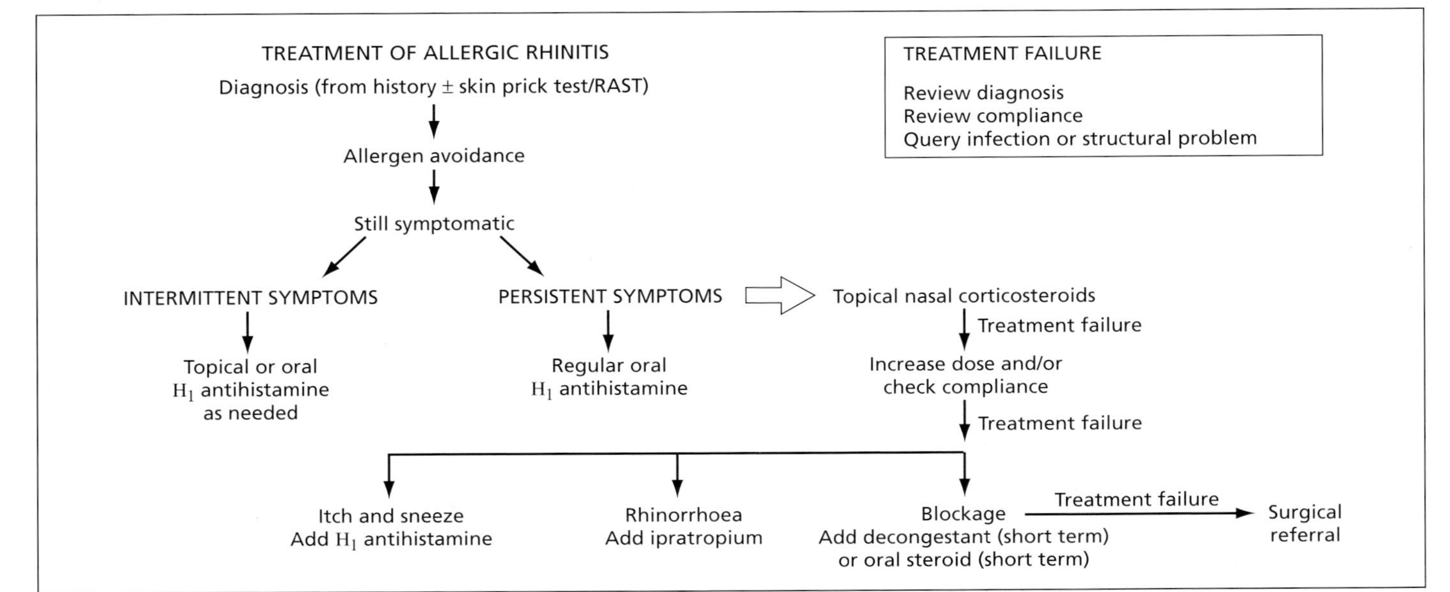

TREATMENT OF ALLERGIC RHINITIS
Diagnosis (from history ± skin prick test/RAST)
Allergen avoidance
Still symptomatic
INTERMITTENT SYMPTOMS
PERSISTENT SYMPTOMS
Topical nasal corticosteroids
Treatment failure
Topical or oral
H_1 antihistamine
as needed
Regular oral
H_1 antihistamine
Increase dose and/or
check compliance
Treatment failure
Itch and sneeze
Add H_1 antihistamine
Rhinorrhoea
Add ipratropium
Blockage
Add decongestant (short term)
or oral steroid (short term)
Treatment failure
Surgical referral
TREATMENT FAILURE
Review diagnosis
Review compliance
Query infection or structural problem

Rhinitis
Management Guidelines

Devised by the British Society for Allergy and Clinical Immunology ENT Sub-Committee

Dr Glenis K. Scadding
Mr Adrian Drake-Lee
Professor Stephen Durham
Dr Peter Howarth
Professor Nicholas Jones
Mr Douglas MacMillan
Dr Rita Mirakian

© Martin Dunitz 2000

Published in the United Kingdom by
Martin Dunitz Ltd
The Livery House
7–9 Pratt Street
London NW1 0AE

ISBN: 1-85317-969-8

Contents

Classification and differential diagnosis

Introduction

Nasal symptoms are often demeaned but their prevalence and effect on the quality of life justify a thoughtful and rational approach, especially in view of the recent observations on the frequent co-existence of rhinitis and asthma, with rhinitis appearing first in 45% of patients, and the fact that adequate nasal treatment can improve pulmonary function.

Everyone is familiar with the symptoms of an occasional viral rhinitis, but prolonged problems such as nasal obstruction, rhinorrhoea or sneezing for at least an hour a day for more than 2 weeks, or secondary effects such as facial pain, loss of sense of smell and postnasal catarrh require diagnosis and treatment.

> *Rhinitis affects 1 in 6 people*
> *Rhinitis affects 1 in 4 adolescents*

WHAT IS RHINITIS?

Blockage	} 2 of 3 symptoms
Running	} for > 1hr/day
(including post nasal drip)	} for > 2 weeks
Sneezing	}
(including nasal itch)	

The number of consultations in general practice for seasonal rhinitis has increased at least fourfold since the 1950s. Allergic rhinitis is now the commonest immunological disorder and the commonest chronic disease of man. Some affected individuals are predisposed to secondary problems such as sinus infection and disturbed sleep. Recent advances in the investigation of nasal symptoms, such as rigid nasal endoscopy and CT scans, have increased the appreciation of the extent of the mucosal abnormality in rhinitis.

Nasal problems are often multifactorial

Confusion in terminology has led to difficulties in comparing the value of different treatments and in analysing aetiology and pathophysiology of rhinitis. The classification shown (Figure 1) defines what remains poorly understood and categorises what is well established.

Nasal problems are often multifactorial and this has to be taken into account when using the classification or considering treatment. For example, a patient with allergic rhinitis may have mucosal oedema obstructing sinus drainage: the mucostasis may predispose the sinuses to bacterial infection. This may occur more readily in those with abnormalities of nasal structure. Treatment which addresses only the acute problem (i.e. a short course of antibiotics) may result in incomplete resolution of the infection or a later recurrence. Since the mucosa of the nose and sinuses is continuous, rhinitis should be called rhinosinusitis.

Figure 1: CLASSIFICATION OF RHINITIS

COMMON FORMS		RARER FORMS	
ALLERGIC	INFECTIVE	OTHER	PART OF SYSTEMIC DISORDER

Seasonal
Perennial
Occupational
	Acute
	Chronic
		Idiopathic
		NARES (non-allergic rhinitis with eosinophilia)
		Drug-induced:
		  • β-blockers
		  • Oral contraceptive
		  • Aspirin
		  • Non-steroidal anti-inflammatory drugs
		  • Local decongestants
		Autonomic (responds to anti-cholinergics)
		Atrophic
		Neoplastic
			Primary defect in mucus
			  • Cystic fibrosis
			  • Young's syndrome
			Primary ciliary dyskinesia
			  • Kartagener's syndrome
			Immunological
			  • Systemic lupus erythematosus
			  • Rheumatoid arthritis
			Acquired immune deficiency syndrome (AIDS)
			Antibody deficiency
			Granulomatous disease
			  • Wegener's
			  • Sarcoidosis
			Hormonal
			  • Hypothyroidism
			  • Pregnancy
			  • Old man's drip

Diagnosis of rhinitis

(a) Taking a history

SYMPTOMS: **Obstructed or blocked?**	SUGGESTED INVESTIGATION:

Often due to rhinitis:

■ This may be clearly seasonal and allergic; however, 60% of patients with a blocked nose all the year around also have an allergic rhinitis which is maintained during winter months by house dust mite allergy.

Nasal examination

■ There may be a co-existing infective element as the hypertrophied allergic mucosa will obstruct sinus ostia and predispose to infection.

Skin prick tests

■ Nasal blockage can be a symptom of mucosal atrophy/dryness or of chronic ethmoidal infection, even when the nasal airway is patent.

Airway tests, e.g. spatula misting, nasal and inspiratory peak flow

SYMPTOMS:
Blocked one side or alternating from side to side?

■ Unilateral obstruction is usually caused by a mechanical obstruction such as septal deviation.

As above

■ Obstruction alternating from side to side indicates a generalised rhinitis which has made the normal 'nasal cycle' more apparent.

SYMPTOMS:
Post nasal drip

■ Green mucopus implies infection but yellow discoloration may be due to eosinophils and allergy.

Nasal smear, skin prick test and referral for endoscopy and CT scan if persistent despite intervention

SYMPTOMS:
Sneezing

■ Common in allergic rhinitis.

Skin prick test

■ Co-existing symptoms of itchy eyes or a tingling palate would make a diagnosis of allergy more likely.

■ Consider the possibility of co-existing asthma.

Peak flow

SYMPTOMS:
Loss of sense of smell

Ask if this is TOTAL or not:

■ Malingerers often deny being able to smell petrol fumes or ammonia. However, these are sensed by the trigeminal nerve, which is unaffected by rhinitis.

■ Partial loss of smell makes it likely there is no significant damage to the olfactory nerve

Refer for formal tests of taste and smell

and that the primary problem is rhinitis, which is potentially treatable, as is anosmia due to nasal polyps.

SYMPTOMS:
Facial pain and pressure

■ Is this exacerbated by upper respiratory tract infections or relieved by the appropriate medical nasal treatment (for allergy and/or infection)? If not, be suspicious that this may not be of nasal origin.

■ Do not forget the many other causes of facial pain e.g. migraine, referred dental pain, tension headaches.

SYMPTOMS:
Runny nose

■ Usually due to an acute upper respiratory tract infection and short lived, or to an allergic rhinitis. If it occurs without any other nasal symptoms it may be due to parasympathetic overactivity.

■ Unilateral nasal discharge in a child is usually due to a foreign body (often foam).

■ Bloody unilateral discharge in an adult – exclude malignancy.

Consider referral for endoscopy/CT scan in patients not responding to simple measures and those with unilateral problems or sero-sanguinous discharge

Referral for endoscopy

Referral for CT scan

Nasal smear

Examination may need anaesthetic

Referral for CT scan

SYMPTOMS:
Vestibulitis

- Staphylococcal infection, often due to plucking of nasal hair and/or nose picking.

SYMPTOMS:
Crusting

- In the vestibule is usually infective (see vestibulitis above).

- Crusting higher in the nasal cavity is an unusual symptom and warrants both a detailed enquiry and inspection. It can occur with a nasal septal perforation of any cause or as a result of nasal involvement in systemic disorders such as sarcoidosis or Wegener's granulomatosis.

SYMPTOMS:
Bleeding

- 90% of the time this derives from a vessel on Little's area and is caused by picking, drying over a septal spur, local corticosteroids, or arises spontaneously without any obvious cause.

- If associated with a unilateral mucopurulent discharge, malignancy needs to be excluded.

*ESR
Referral for
special tests
and/or biopsy
(urgent if ESR
high)*

Referral

OTHER DETAILS

In Britain it is not uncommon for patients who are dissatisfied with the appearance of their nose to present with other nasal symptoms.

Onset

SUGGESTED INVESTIGATION:

■ Did symptoms follow an upper respiratory tract infection which never resolved? This may imply a residue of ethmoidal infection which has not cleared.

Referral for possible CT scan if no response to antibiotics, decongestants or topical steroids

■ Are symptoms seasonal or initiated by any factors e.g. dusting, occupation, animals?

Skin prick test

Previous Medication

■ Ask what has been tried and HOW and FOR HOW LONG.

■ 75% of patients with rhinitis failing to respond to medical treatment have taken their spray or drops incorrectly or not for long enough or have not been advised about regular use.

■ Ask about decongestant use and systemic medication.

■ In sinusitis not responding to antibiotics consider an anaerobic or fungal infection.

Recurrent infection

■ In patients with recurrent or unusual infections consider testing.

Previous Surgery or Trauma

■ Patients who have had surgery directed at their maxillary sinuses without improvement may have persistent ethmoidal disease.

Family History

■ Allergic rhinitis is often associated with atopy (asthma, eczema, hay fever) in other family members.

Medical History

■ A history of bronchiectasis may indicate a disorder of ciliary motility which affects the sinuses.

■ Past or present asthma, eczema, or hay fever make it almost certain that allergic rhinitis is contributing to the symptoms.

SUGGESTED INVESTIGATION: *Immune function (see blood tests on p. 14), nasal mucociliary clearance*

Referral for CT scan

Ciliary beat frequency

(b) Nasal Examination

External appearance

■ A deviated septum can sometimes be apparent externally.

■ Systemic disorders can affect the external appearance e.g. the painless erythema and swelling of the nose which may be seen in sarcoid.

■ Nasal ulceration warrants referral for biopsy.

■ Gross nasal polyps may produce expansion of the nasal bones.

■ A crease (a horizontal crease above the tip of the nose) is characteristic of a marked allergic rhinitis due to the patient persistently rubbing their nose.

Airflow

■ Ask the patient to breathe normally and hold a cold metal spatula or mirror under the nostrils to see the extent of misting.

Anterior nares

■ Gently lift back the tip of the nose; this is painless and particularly useful in children. It can show an anterior deviation of the septum, narrowing of the nasal valve and inferior turbinate hypertrophy.

Nasal airway

■ While a headlight and a Thudichum's speculum are helpful, a good view can be obtained using an auriscope. Ask the patient to breathe through their mouth in order to avoid misting of the lens.

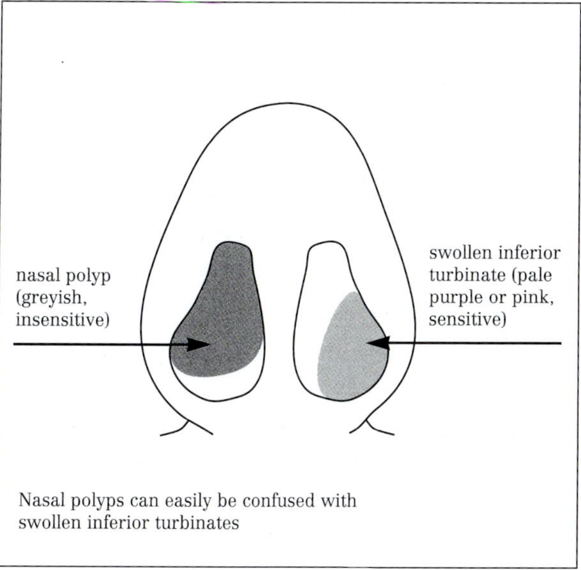

Nasal polyps can easily be confused with swollen inferior turbinates

■ Unilateral nasal polyps should be referred for biopsy to exclude malignancy.

■ Polyps are rare in children except when associated with cystic fibrosis.

Secretions

■ Secretions are found in a wide variety of conditions ranging from immune deficiencies and allergy through to chronic sinusitis.

■ Pus under the middle turbinate is a sign of ethmoidal or maxillary sinusitis. Yellow mucus is not always infected and may be due to eosinophils.

Postnasal space

■ Mucopus may be seen tracking down the back of the pharynx and may cause pharyngitis.

■ Occasionally a unilateral, large single antrochoanal polyp may be seen.

Palpation

■ Tenderness under the supraorbital rim is characteristic of acute frontal sinusitis.

■ Swelling of the cheek is normally of dental origin and is rare in maxillary sinusitis.

■ Periorbital swelling with a sinus infection (periorbital cellulitis) is serious and justifies an urgent referral.

Endoscopes

Both rigid and flexible endoscopes have greatly helped in the diagnosis of sinus problems particularly when medical treatment has failed. They help detect ethmoidal infection and anatomical abnormalities. Their use is largely confined to specialist clinics at present.

(c) Skin Prick Tests

Serious reactions to skin prick tests are exceedingly rare provided that:

■ patients with a history of anaphylaxis are excluded

■ subcutaneous or intradermal testing is avoided.

Skin prick testing for common aeroallergens can be performed in a GP surgery by a trained operator (e.g. allergy nurse).

A few test substances will diagnose the majority of allergic rhinitis patients:

■ House dust mites

■ Grass pollen

■ Cat dander

■ Dog dander

■ A negative control (saline)

■ A positive control (histamine)

Record the weal from each substance – reactions 3mm in diameter greater than the negative control are regarded as positive, although in children smaller weals may be significant.

RAST/IgE

Under these circumstances blood can be sent from radioallergosorbent (RAST) testing, either looking for single specific sensitivities or employing a screen of several likely allergens. Measurements of total serum IgE are not generally helpful in rhinitis since this is raised in only 50% of patients despite a raised specific IgE – exceptions to this are children and the elderly, where this measurement can be helpful.

Nasal tests

Negative skin prick tests mean that a diagnosis of allergic rhinitis is unlikely, but not impossible. In specialised centres, tests such as nasal smears for eosinophils and nasal allergen challenge can be undertaken.

Blood tests

In patients with recurrent infections consider checking full blood count, ESR, serum immunoglobulins, urea, electrolytes, liver function tests, blood sugar and urine sugar. Consider referral for tests of mucociliary function.

(d) Other Investigations

Plain sinus X-rays

■ Plain sinus X-rays have a limited place in the investigation of rhinosinusitis. They fail to detect ethmoidal disease and even when they are abnormal they do not help in defining the cause of the problem.

■ They do have a role in acute sinusitis which has failed to respond to 36 hours of antibiotics and decongestants. An opaque antrum under these conditions indicates that a sinus washout may be needed.

Treat the patient and not the X-rays

Computerised tomography

■ A CT scan should not be used as a 'screening investigation'.

■ Its place is in patients who have failed to respond to medical treatment and whose history and examination is suggestive of ethmoidal infection or in those in whom malignancy is suspected; it is carried out prior to surgery in order to define the anatomy and the extent of their disease.

Treatment of rhinitis

(a) Allergen Avoidance Measures

Management of patients with rhinitis symptoms should always include identification and, where possible, avoidance of causal factors. The commonest cause of perennial allergic rhinitis symptoms are sensitivity to house dust mite and domestic pets. Important seasonal causes include allergy to pollens (tree pollen in springtime, grass and weeds during the summer) and mould spores during the late summer and autumn months.

Occupational allergens may provoke perennial symptoms. It is therefore essential to ask whether symptoms are work-related i.e. occur during the week or during the evenings after work, and improve at weekends and whilst on holiday.

A careful drug history should always be taken (see Table 1 for likely sources of drug allergy).

Table 1: AVOIDANCE OF IDENTIFIABLE CAUSE

Aeroallergens

Perennial:	House dust mite, cats, dogs
Seasonal:	Tree and grass pollen, mould spores

Occupational

Biological:	Flour, laboratory animals, latex, etc.
Chemical:	Low molecular weight substances e.g. isocyanates, acid anhydrides, colophony etc.

Drugs

Aspirin, NSAIDs, antihypertensives, oral contraceptive pill, hormone replacement therapy.

Food allergy may occasionally provoke rhinitis. Almost invariably this rare association is accompanied by other manifestations of allergy such as oral and/or gastro-intestinal symptoms, rash or, occasionally, anaphylaxis.

House Dust Mite Avoidance

The major allergen in house dust mite (Der pI) has now been identified, cloned and sequenced. House dust mites are found in mattresses, pillows, bedcovers, carpets (particularly wool) and soft furnishing throughout the home. Optimal conditions for mite growth are achieved through well insulated, centrally heated homes!

Mattress/bedding barrier intervention has been shown to reduce mite allergen exposure and improve clinical symptoms of both asthma and rhinitis.

Acaricides kill mites but do not eliminate the allergen and so their use has to be accompanied by vigorous vacuuming. Such an approach has been shown to be beneficial in rhinitis. An alternative is the use of denaturing agents, such as tannic acid, that destroy the allergen. This has not been tested in rhinitis.

The BSACI Position Paper (Colloff et al 1992) recommends use of bedding barrier intervention, regular vacuuming of carpets and soft furnishings and, where possible, use of alternative cork, vinyl or hardwood floors.

Table 2: HOUSE DUST MITE AVOIDANCE

- Mattress covers
- Covers for pillows and bedding
- Liquid nitrogen
- Acaricides, protein denaturing agents
- Regulation of ventilation, humidity of home
- Minimise soft furnishings/toys in bedroom
- Vacuuming

Animal Allergens

The major cat allergen (Fel dI) is a salivary protein which is preened on to the fur where it dries into flakes. These become airborne as minute (<2.5 μm) particles which remain airborne for many hours and are very respirable.

Families with atopic members should be advised against having furred animals in the home. Psychosocial factors may render dogmatic statements about removal of a family pet unwise. In such circumstances advice may be ignored and the doctor-patient relationship embarrassed.

Where removal of a pet is not possible, advice can be given to confine the animal outside or to the kitchen. Patients should be advised that vigorous, prolonged cleaning measures are required in order to satisfactorily reduce allergen levels.

Recent studies have suggested that washing the cat at least once weekly when combined with other cleaning measures plus the use of HEPA filters may effectively reduce airborne cat allergen levels in the home. Families may be advised that an animal should not be replaced.

Cat allergen may remain in the home for many months after removal of a pet.

Grass Pollen Avoidance

Avoidance of pollens is frequently not possible. However, simple advice includes keeping windows shut in cars and buildings. Wearing sunglasses may reduce eye symptoms. Certain cars nowadays are fitted with pollen filters.

Patients should be advised to avoid walking in open grassy spaces, particularly during the early morning, evening and at night when pollen counts are at their highest.

If affordable, a holiday by the sea or abroad during the peak pollen season may be recommended.

(b) Pharmacotherapy

Introduction

Patients need drugs for allergic rhinitis if avoiding the allergen is impossible or fails to control symptoms.

In recent years, the mainstay of treatment for allergic rhinitis has been the use of topical corticosteroid nasal sprays and the newer non-sedating antihistamines. These may be highly effective when used either alone or in combination. Topical sodium cromoglycate represents an alternative but weaker anti-inflammatory agent to corticosteroids, particularly in young children. Topical anticholinergic drugs and decongestants may have a part to play in defined circumstances.

Corticosteroids and sodium cromoglycate affect the underlying allergic process and should be used as first line treatment for most patients. Decongestants simply relieve symptoms, and antihistamines have weak anti-inflammatory activity – symptomatic relief of sneezing, running and itching is their major effect.

Anti-allergy Drugs

Patients should start to take these before exposure to seasonal allergen begins.

Corticosteroids: Topical corticosteroids are highly effective against all nasal symptoms, including nasal congestion and blockage, in the majority of sufferers. Beclomethasone dipropionate, budesonide, flunisolide, triamcinolone acetonide, fluticasone propionate and mometasone furoate are available in aqueous formulations. Side effects are minor and include local irritation (in 5–10% of patients) and light bleeding. A retrospective study suggests that use of intranasal steroids does not increase the risk of cataract or glaucoma. Septal perforation is exceedingly rare as a result of local steroid use. Fluticasone propionate and mometasone furoate, which are effective once daily, have low bioavailability. Fluticasone propionate is the only topical corticosteroid licensed for use in children as young as 4.

The commonest reason for treatment failure with topical corticosteroids is that the medication has not been taken regularly, even in the absence of symptoms. For maximal effect in seasonal rhinitis the drug should be commenced before the season. Systemic effects are rare at conventional doses, although care should be exercised when concomitant corticosteroids are used for asthma and/or eczema. Growth suppression in children has been noted with budesonide at 400 µg daily and with beclomethasone dipropionate 168 µg twice daily when used regularly over 1 year, but not with mometasone furoate 100 µg daily. There are as yet few data on nasal absorption of different topical corticosteroids, and long-term safety data on each are awaited. It makes sense at present to use preparations with the least oral bioavailability and to monitor growth in all children receiving topical nasal corticosteroids. There are some patients who appear to be particularly sensitive to systemic effects. The dose should be kept as small as possible and used once daily in the morning. In smaller children non-steroidal medication could be substituted once control is achieved.

Systemic corticosteroids: Short courses of oral corticosteroids may be needed for severe symptoms, for example when pollen levels are high or when blockage is so severe that nasal sprays are ineffective. Patients with no contra-indications should take the minimum effective dose, for no more than 2 weeks (20mg of prednisolone daily for 5 days is often helpful), and should continue with intranasal therapy.

Depot intramuscular corticosteroids are not recommended, as the dose is not controllable and local and systemic side-effects can occur. It is better to give patients maximal intranasal corticosteroids and regular antihistamine, before and during the pollen season, with a supply of oral corticosteroids to use on special occasions or when the pollen count is particularly high.

Betamethasone nose drops used in the head down and forward position relieve allergic swelling in the middle meatal region, and can help nasal polyposis. Combined with oral corticosteroids (30mg prednisolone over 5 days), a 2 week course of betamethasone can shrink nasal polyps. Patients commonly overuse them, as the drops are not metered. Short-term use at the beginning of treatment or during exacerbations is best. Fluticasone propionate is now available in a metered drop formulation (nasules) and is effective in the treatment of nasal polyposis.

Sodium cromoglycate: To be effective in prophylaxis, sodium cromoglycate needs to be taken four times a day. It is available as insufflation, drops or spray. We do not recommend combinations with xylometazoline.

Cromoglycate is well tolerated, although it can be an irritant initially. It is partially effective against all symptoms of rhinitis with no greater effect than H_1 antihistamines, but it is an option in young children.

Cromoglycate eye drops help in the prophylaxis of allergic conjunctivitis.

Symptomatic Relief

Antihistamines

Antihistamines are particularly effective for symptoms of sneezing, itching and watery rhinorrhoea although, unlike topical corticosteroids, they have little effect on nasal blockage. However, antihistamines have the advantage of being additionally effective for eye, palatal and throat symptoms. Furthermore, some patients prefer the convenience of a once or twice daily oral preparation to the use of sprays.

The newer antihistamines produce less sedation and psychomotor impairment than the older drugs and are equally effective.

Non-sedative antihistamines include acrivastine, loratadine, cetirizine, fexofenadine and mizolastine. All have been shown to be effective in placebo-controlled trials of seasonal and perennial allergic rhinitis. Ideally all should be avoided during pregnancy.

Prolongation of the QT interval on ECG and occasional incidences of ventricular arrhythmias (torsades de pointes) have been reported with terfenadine and astemizole (the latter now withdrawn). Underlying factors were excessive dose, hepatic impairment and concomitant use of ketoconazole, erythromycin-type drugs or grapefruit juice, which modify hepatic metabolism. Patients with a congenitally prolonged QT interval were at risk, as also were those with other cardiac problems and hypokalaemia. Although most other antihistamines appear safer in this regard, QT prolongation has been reported at high doses of azelastine and ebastine. Excessive doses should not be used. In patients with the above predisposing factors it is probably safest to use a non-hepatically metabolised drug such as cetirizine or fexofenadine.

Ketotifen has both antihistamine and cromoglycate-like effects and is useful in small children who find using nasal sprays and drops difficult. However, sedation can be a problem.

Two topical nasal antihistamines azelastine and levocabastine are effective, but occasional patients note local irritation or an unpleasant taste.

Adding an H_2 blocker may help patients who do not respond to full doses of H_1 blockers.

Decongestants

Systemic decongestants are of doubtful value. They can cause hyperactivity in children, and can raise blood pressure. Local decongestants are useful, for example, at the start of therapy with inhaled corticosteroids, or before an aeroplane flight; prolonged use (more than a week) carries a danger of rebound nasal blockage and rhinitis medicamentosa.

Ipratropium bromide

Intranasal ipratropium bromide helps patients with watery rhinorrhoea only. Several doses should be taken when symptoms are worse – usually early morning – and only one or two doses taken later in the day in order to control symptoms without producing excessive nasal dryness. Prolonged use occasionally produces complete remission.

Leukotriene receptor antagonists

These have a moderate effect, mainly against obstruction and mucus production in rhinitis trials. Their major place is likely to be in aspirin-sensitive nasal polyposis, in which leukotriene overproduction and exquisite sensitivity occur.

Table 3: EFFECTS OF VARIOUS DRUGS ON SYMPTOMS OF ALLERGIC RHINITIS

	Itching/ sneezing	Discharge	Blockage	Anosmia
Cromoglycate	++	+	+	-
Decongestant	-	-	+++	-
Antihistamine	++	++	+/-	-
Ipratropium	-	++	-	-
Topical steroids	+++	+++	+++	+
Oral steroids	+++	+++	+++	++

After N. Mygind 1992, Rhinology. Surgical Supplement

Summary

Pharmacotherapy should always be combined with allergen avoidance measures where possible. Careful attention should be paid in the history to the type and dominance of the patient's symptoms and drugs used alone or in combination to match the patient's symptom profile (Table 3).

The importance of regular prophylactic medication, even in the absence of symptoms, requires emphasis. Treatment failure should always provoke a review of compliance.

If regular treatment has been unsuccessful, then the diagnosis should be reviewed, and the need for alternative treatment (e.g. surgery for polyps or septal deviation) or, where appropriate in selected patients, the need for allergen-specific immunotherapy should be re-assessed.

(c) Immunotherapy

Both seasonal and perennial allergic rhinitis may
be effectively managed with a combination of
allergen avoidance measures plus topical
corticosteroids and oral non-sedating
antihistamines. There remains a group of subjects
who, despite regular use of medication, continue to
have marked symptoms. It is for pollen-sensitive
patients who fail to respond to conventional
pharmacotherapy that allergen injection
immunotherapy is indicated.

Indications

Subjects should give a clear history of seasonal
symptoms, a positive skin prick test and/or raised
allergen specific IgE concentrations to grass pollen,
and a history of poor symptom control with
conventional anti-allergic drugs.

Patients with multiple allergies and other
immunological or medical disease are excluded. In
the United Kingdom, patients with chronic asthma,
even mild disease, are also excluded. Seasonal
asthma is not a contraindication provided that the
patient is asymptomatic outside the pollen season.

Mechanism of Immunotherapy

Recent research suggests that immunotherapy may
act by inducing immune deviation of T-lymphocyte
responses (TH_2 to TH_1) or by inducing T-
lymphocyte unresponsiveness (anergy).

Efficacy

The efficacy of immunotherapy in seasonal allergic
rhinitis (grass pollen, ragweed and birch) has been
confirmed in a number of carefully controlled
clinical studies. Although immunotherapy may be
effective in patients with perennial allergy due to
house dust mite and animal danders, at present it

is available in the United Kingdom only in a few
specialised centres.

Allergen injection immunotherapy represents a
specific treatment for allergic disease and, unlike
conventional pharmacological treatment, has the
potential to alter the course of allergic disease. For
example, in carefully selected patients, 3 years of
grass pollen immunotherapy provided long-term
benefit for at least 3 years after discontinuation.

Safety

In 1986, the Committee on Safety of Medicines
expressed concern about a number of deaths (25
reported over 30 years) from severe bronchospasm
and anaphylaxis; these deaths were almost
exclusively confined to patients with asthma.
Allergen injection immunotherapy should be given
where facilities for resuscitation are available and
patients should be kept under medical observation
for at least 1 hour after injections. Patients with
chronic asthma are specifically excluded. This
post-injection observation interval (unlike the
30 minutes recommended in USA and Europe) has
made immunotherapy impracticable for both
physicians and patients in the United Kingdom at
present, except in specialised centres.

Alternative routes

Research suggests that sublingual, intranasal or
oral immunotherapy may prove effective. Further
studies are in progress.

(d) The Place of Surgery

The treatment of rhinitis is essentially medical with surgical help in selected cases for relief of obstruction or when medical treatment is not fully effective.

The role of surgery is difficult to place for, in some conditions, such as nasal polyps, it has a major role in symptomatic control and in others, such as sarcoid, it has very little place except in reconstruction. In general, minimal surgery should be used in these patients and surgery can be used for diagnosis (nasal biopsy), for improving nasal function and for correction of anatomical deformity.

Improving Nasal Function

The nose may be blocked by polyps, septal deviation, large inferior turbinates and adhesions. Although nasal polyps may respond to corticosteroids, those that do not can be removed by a number of methods including simple snares and forceps under direct vision. More recently rigid endoscopes have been used to help view the middle meatus and ethmoid sinuses in greater detail and surgery can be performed in the nose using these (functional endoscopic sinus surgery or FESS).

> *Nasal allergy and infection frequently coexist and can be treated together*

In patients with chronic ethmoiditis where anatomical variations in the middle meatus cause localised disease by obstructing sinus drainage, functional endoscopic sinus surgery is frequently beneficial. Surgery may be required to the septum or turbinates in allergic rhinitis to allow the ingress of nasal sprays.

Correction of Cosmetic Deformity

This may be corrected by the operation of septorhinoplasty.

Paediatric rhinitis

Rhinitis in toddlers is frequently due to upper respiratory tract infections, normal children having 6 to 8 per year. However, it can be allergic and is often then associated with other atopic manifestations such as eczema. A persistent unilateral purulent discharge may indicate a foreign body (often foam). Chronic bilateral purulent rhinorrhoea may be a manifestation of underlying immune abnormalities such as defective mucociliary clearance or immunoglobulin deficiency. Developmental abnormalities such as choanal atresia or encephalocoele present with nasal obstruction and discharge. Therefore, in children not responding to simple treatments, ENT referral is advisable.

Nasal polyps are rare in childhood and if present a sweat test should be undertaken to check for cystic fibrosis. Epistaxis is not uncommon in allergic rhinitis since the nose is itchy and boggy and is often picked or scratched.

Treatment for allergic rhinitis in small children depends mainly on allergen avoidance and it is in this age group that dietary factors such as milk may be relevant. However, this will almost always be associated with other immediate features of food allergy such as rash or oral itching and swelling. Food allergy only very rarely causes symptoms confined to one organ. A trial of a dairy-free diet (given with calcium supplementation) followed by dairy reintroduction may confirm a diagnosis, but dietetic help should be sought.

Few drug treatments are available. Under the age of 2, nasal saline drops or sprays can help to clear the nose before eating. Sodium cromoglycate is the main anti-inflammatory available at present for children under the age of 4 years. Frequent use can be aided by the advice to put the spray on the table and to administer it before meals. Fluticasone dipropionate is available for children of 4 years and over and has the advantage of once-daily usage so that the spray can be put in when the child is asleep if there is great aversion to nasal therapy. Oral therapy with ketotifen syrup is available for children of 2 years upwards. Other antihistamine availability is as shown. Topical corticosteroids may cause minor bleeding especially if used with poor technique so that the spray lands on the septum.

Drug Treatment of Allergic Rhinitis in Children

Prophylaxis:

- Sodium cromoglycate or one of the following:

  Fluticasone propionate (age > 4 years)
  Flunisolide (age > 5 years)
  Beclomethasone dipropionate (age > 6 years)
  Triamcinolone acetonide (age > 6 years)
  Mometasone furonate (age > 6 years)

Relief:

- Antihistamines (local)

  Azelastine (age > 5 years)
  Levocabastine (age > 5 years)

- Antihistamines (oral)

  Cetirizine (sugar-free syrup)
  - 5mg daily (age 2-6 years)
  - 10mg daily (age > 6 years)
  Loratadine
  - 5mg daily (bodyweight < 30kg,
    age 2-12 years)
  - 10mg daily (bodyweight > 30kg)
  Terfenadine (sugar-free syrup)*
  - 15mg twice daily (age 3-6 years)
  - 30mg twice daily (age 6-12 years)

- *Sedating antihistamines impair academic performance and should be avoided.*

** See special precautions that apply to this drug.*

Asthma and rhinitis

Many asthmatics (66% to 80%) also have rhinitis. Rhinitis itself is a risk factor for the development of asthma and exacerbations caused by seasonal pollen or by allergen challenge are associated with the development of bronchial hyper-reactivity. Viral rhinitis is a frequent precipitant of asthmatic attacks.

In several studies the treatment of rhinitis has been shown to improve concomitant asthma. In one 400 µg of beclomethasone dipropionate was more effective at decreasing bronchial hyper-reactivity when used nasally than when inhaled! Chronic rhinosinusitis with or without nasal polyposis may be associated with asthma that is severe and requires frequent courses of oral corticosteroids. These may not only improve asthma but also can decrease polyp size and may obviate the need for surgery or improve surgical access. Surgical treatment improves not only nasal symptoms but also the asthma. In a retrospective study it decreased hospitalisation and the need for oral steroids. Controlled trials are needed to test this. However, there is no evidence that a nasal polypectomy worsens asthma or causes its development.

Rhinitis in pregnancy

In allergic rhinitis allergen avoidance is important both to decrease the need for medication and as a protective measure since the offspring have a greater than 30% chance of being atopic. The risk/benefit ratio of any drug therapy must be carefully considered since none of the medications used have been definitively proven to lack foetal effects. Some antihistamines may increase the risk of spontaneous abortion or congenital malformation, but topical corticosteroids have shown no evidence of harmful effects. There has been no danger associated with sodium cromoglycate during pregnancy.

The rhinitis of pregnancy, which is thought to be similar with that associated with oral contraceptives and hormone replacement therapy, can be quite distressing especially at night when sleep is difficult. The sparing use of topical vasoconstrictors has been suggested; however, a recent report suggests that this could be a risk factor for abdominal malformation. The use of nasal douching or a nasal saline spray may be effective. Reassurance that this is a self-limiting condition may be the only therapy necessary.

Occupational rhinitis

Occupational rhinitis is induced by an agent inhaled at work. It is common but generally under-reported. It may occur alone but it is frequently associated with asthma. High molecular weight proteins can be responsible by acting as allergens and by inducing a classical IgE mediated Type 1 reaction while low molecular weight chemicals can act both as haptens and by a non-IgE dependent mechanism. Occupational rhinitis occurs before asthma for high molecular weight agents.

Sensitising agents typically have a latent interval between the exposure and the onset of the symptoms. Irritants may act with an 'adjuvant' effect which causes injury to the upper airway mucosa facilitating sensitisation. Predisposing factors are an atopic predisposition, viral infections and environmental irritants such as smoking, sulphur dioxide, nitrogen dioxide, ozone, ammonia, etc. The most common causes of occupational rhinitis are shown in Table 4.

The clinical history is very important, as symptoms occur after a working day and improve during the weekend and during the holidays. Only occasionally are skin tests or RAST helpful in diagnosis (usually in cases of allergy to laboratory animals, flour or penicillin), and therefore nasal provocation tests may be indicated. Patients need to complete a 2–4 week chart of symptoms. Once the diagnosis is established, the patient should be removed from further exposure. It is important that preventative measures are taken by the use of protective clothes, gloves and masks in 'at-risk' occupations.

Table 4: MOST COMMON CAUSES OF OCCUPATIONAL RHINITIS

AGENTS	HMW	LMW	INDUSTRY
animal proteins	dandruff, fur, urine, droppings		laboratory, breeding
vegetable proteins	grain/flour latex		food processing, bakers, hospital workers
enzymes (from animal and vegetable sources)	papain, amylase, trypsin, cellulose etc		manufacture, food processing, detergents, pharmaceuticals
microbial agents	antibiotics		manufacture
chemicals		isocyanates pinewood resins (colophony) acid anhydrides	plastic/paint soldering (electric trade)/ glue epoxy resins

Conclusions

Rhinitis is a common condition. It is frequently allergic and found in co-existence with asthma. General Practitioners are ideally placed to diagnose and treat the majority of allergic rhinitis sufferers, with Consultant referral for those who fail to respond. Successful treatment may improve concomitant asthma, possibly by restoring normal nasal filtration and humidification functions. It remains to be seen whether treatment of isolated rhinitis can delay or prevent the development of asthma in predisposed individuals.

ENT referral is also needed for unilateral nasal problems, nasal perforations, ulceration or collapse, sero-sanguineous discharge, crusting high in the nasal cavity and recurrent infections. It is needed urgently for periorbital cellulitis.

Further reading

Bousquet J, van Cauwenberge P, Bachert C *et al.* Allergic rhinitis and its impact on asthma (ARIA). WHO position paper (in press) 2000.

Colloff MJ, Ayres J, Carswell PH *et al.* The control of allergens of dust mites and domestic pets. A position paper. *Clin Exp Allergy* 1992; **22**: 1–28.

Durham SR, ed. *ABC of Allergies.* London: BMA; 1998.

Durham SR, Walker SM, Varga EM *et al.* Long-term clinical efficacy of grass pollen immunotherapy. *N Engl J Med* 1999; **341**: 468–475.

Scadding GK, Durham SR. Immunology of the nasal mucosa. In: Jones AS, Phillips DE, Hilgers FJM, eds. *Diseases of the Head and Neck, Nose and Throat.* London: Arnold; 1997.

Scadding GK, Mygind N. *Fast Facts: Allergic Rhinitis.* Oxford: Health Press; 2000.

Schenkel EJ, Skoner DP, Bronsky EA *et al.* Absence of growth retardation in children with perennial allergic rhinitis following 1 year of treatment with mometasone furoate aqueous nasal spray. *Paediatrics* 2000; **105**(2): electronic 22.

Skoner DP, Rachelefsky GS, Meltzer EO *et al.* Detection of growth suppression in children during treatment with intranasal beclomethasone dipropionate. *Paediatrics* 2000; **105**(2): electronic 23.

Weiner JM, Abramson MJ, Puy RM. Intranasal corticosteroids versus oral H1 receptor antagonists in allergic rhinitis: systemic review of randomised control trials. *BMJ* 1998; **317**: 1624–1629.

Wolthers OD, Pedersen S. Short-term growth in children with allergic rhinitis treated with oral antihistamine, depot and intranasal glucocorticosteroids. *Acta Paediatr* 1993; **82**: 635–640.

Index